Hèla Ben Jmaà
Rim Karray
Emna Ketata

Post-traumatic aortic dissections

Hèla Ben Jmaà
Rim Karray
Emna Ketata

Post-traumatic aortic dissections

Aortic trauma

ScienciaScripts

Imprint

Any brand names and product names mentioned in this book are subject to trademark, brand or patent protection and are trademarks or registered trademarks of their respective holders. The use of brand names, product names, common names, trade names, product descriptions etc. even without a particular marking in this work is in no way to be construed to mean that such names may be regarded as unrestricted in respect of trademark and brand protection legislation and could thus be used by anyone.

Cover image: www.ingimage.com

This book is a translation from the original published under ISBN 978-620-6-71568-9.

Publisher:
Sciencia Scripts
is a trademark of
Dodo Books Indian Ocean Ltd. and OmniScriptum S.R.L publishing group

120 High Road, East Finchley, London, N2 9ED, United Kingdom
Str. Armeneasca 28/1, office 1, Chisinau MD-2012, Republic of Moldova, Europe
Printed at: see last page
ISBN: 978-620-7-98381-0

I- LIST OF ABBREVIATIONS

- AIS: Abbreviated Injury Scale
- ALAT: Alanine Amino Transferase
- ASAT: Aspartate Amino Transferase
- AVP: Accidents de la Voie Publique (Public road accidents)
- Thoracic angio-CT: Thoracic angio-modensitometry.
- Body Scanner : Integral body scanner
- CCVT: Cardiovascular and Thoracic Surgery
- ECC: Extracorporeal Circulation
- RBC: Red blood cells
- CT scanner: Computational Tomography.
- DMI: Electronic Medical Record
- ECG: Electrocardiogram
- TEE: Transesophageal echocardiography
- TTE: Trans-Thoracic Ultrasound
- FAST: Focused Assessment with Sonography for Trauma
- HR: Heart Rate
- LVEF: Left Ventricular Ejection Fraction
- RF: Respiratory Rate
- GAD: Glycemia in the Finger
- Glasgow : Glasgow Score
- LMWH: Low Molecular Weight Heparin
- PAH: Pulmonary Arterial Hypertension
- HTIC: Intracranial Hypertension
- PPI: Proton Pump Inhibitors
- ISS: Injury Severity Score
- Mm Hg: millimeter of mercury
- DBP: Diastolic Blood Pressure
- PAS: Systolic Blood Pressure
- PFC: Plasmas, Fresh Frozen
- TTR: Traumatic Aortic Ruptures
- RTIA: Traumatic Aortic Isthmus Rupture
- RTS: Revised Trauma Score
- SAMU: Emergency Medical Service
- SAO2: Mean Oxygen Saturation
- SMUR: Service Mobile d'Urgence et de Réanimation (Mobile emergency and resuscitation service)
- VTE: Endovascular treatment
- PT: Prothrombin rate

- CRT: Cutaneous Recoloration Time
- TRISS: Trauma and Injury Severity Score
- VAS: Voies Aériennes Supérieures (upper airways)

Table of contents

I-   Introduction :

Since the first observations of closed chest trauma in the mid-twentieth century[ème] , progress in the field of traumatology has been considerable. Historically, these injuries, and in particular aortic injuries, have been studied by health professionals, due to their frequency and severity [1]. They are considered to be one of the most serious complications of polytrauma, generally occurring as a result of trauma closed by shear forces. These injuries are typically observed in road accidents or falls from great heights. The most frequent location of these injuries is at the aortic isthmus, a vulnerable point of the aortic arch [2, 3]. The management of aortic trauma requires rapid and rigorous intervention, and is therefore a medical-surgical emergency.

However, despite medical advances, traumatic aortic injury has a pre-hospital survival rate of less than 25% [4, 5]. Moreover, one-third to one-half of patients die shortly after hospital admission [4, 6]. These lesions are among the leading causes of immediate mortality in polytrauma patients, second only to head trauma [7].

Concomitant lesions can also worsen the patient's general condition, posing a challenge for the physician in the initial phase of patient management.

Typically, these lesions are characterized by marked hemodynamic instability, hemorrhagic shock and even loss of consciousness.

Symptoms such as chest pain, paraplegia or dyspnoea may also be observed [8].

In the past, urgent surgical revision by temporary suture, graft interposition or thoracic aortic replacement represented the only therapeutic option. However, this procedure, particularly in polytrauma patients, was associated with a high risk of mortality, reaching up to 42% [9]. Recently, the implantation of a stent graft in the damaged part of the thoracic aorta, an innovative endovascular method known as endovascular thoracic aortic repair, has become the standard of care [10, 11].

An aortic stent graft is a device that acts as a new inner lining for the aorta, helping to redirect blood flow. It is usually composed of a metal frame, often made of nickel-titanium alloy (Nitinol), which provides stability and support once deployed in the aorta [13].

II- Epidemiology of aortic trauma:

The epidemiology of traumatic aortic rupture is difficult to assess. It is often underestimated. Depending on the study, they account for 10 to 16% of traffic accidents [14]. Their relative rarity, despite the frequency of serious accidents, is explained by several factors, notably the high immediate mortality rate and the low number of patients who undergo rapid surgery.

Numbers vary considerably between studies. For example, Cook J's study [15] of 104 patients with traumatic aortic injury and Cheng Y-T's study [16] of 287 patients admitted with traumatic aortic injury noted significantly high numbers.

Table I: Comparative table of published studies and reviews of traumatic aortic injury:

Authors	Period	Workforce
Cook J [15]	Between 1975 and 1990	104
Rousseau H [17]	Between 1981 and 2003	76
Gammié JS [18]	Between January 1988 and June 1997	42
Akouwah E [19]	Between July 2000 and July 2006	15
Denguir R[12]	Between 2000 and 2012	37
Lettinga-van De Poll T [20]	Until January 2006	284
Cheng Y-T [16]	Between January 2004 and December 2013	287
Dinh K [21]	Between January 2010 and December 2019	39
Bae M [22]	Between January 2016 and December 2019	10

Studies conducted on this subject have shown varied demographic characteristics in patients with traumatic aortic lesions. For example, the study by Cook J [15] revealed a mean age of 31 years with a proportion of male patients of 81%, suggesting a prevalence of these lesions in a young, male population. In contrast, the study by Gammie JS [18] was characterized by a female majority (83%) and a mean age of 34 years, highlighting the possibility that young women may also be at risk.

According to research [23], traumatic lesions of the aorta occur in only 0.1-1.0% of children with thoracic trauma, underscoring their rarity in young patients.

Thus, these variations in demographic characteristics suggest potential differences in risk factors and susceptibility related ʊgender and age.

Table II: Summary table of demographic characteristics of aortic trauma :

Authors	Average age (years)	Percentage of men	Percentage of women
Cook J [15]	31 years old	81%	19%
Rousseau H [17]	37 years old	85%	15%
Gammie JS [18]	34 years old	17%	83%
Akouwah E [19]	30 ± 12 years	75%	25%
Denguir R [12]	38 years old	89%	11%
Cheng Y-T [16]	41.66 years old	80,50%	19,50%

In the literature, it is frequently noted that post-traumatic aortic lesions occur in healthy individuals, without notable comorbidities such as hypertension, diabetes or a history of cardiac surgery [24]. This suggests an inherent vulnerability of the aorta to traumatic injury, even in the absence of conventional risk factors.

Similarly, several studies have indicated that although hypertension and atherosclerosis can weaken the aorta and increase the risk of injury in the event of trauma [25], a wide range of patients with no significant medical history remain susceptible to this type of injury.

III- Temporal distribution of traumatic accidents :

Previous research has highlighted the influence of behavioural and environmental factors on the risk and temporal distribution of serious accidents leading to aortic lesions. Among these factors, reduced visibility, increased traffic intensity and the adoption of risky behaviours significantly increase the probability of accidents during certain periods of the day, particularly in the evening [26].

IV- Pathophysiology of post-traumatic aortic damage :
1- Circumstances of accidents:

Traumatic rupture of the aorta, often following severe thoracic trauma, involves several pathophysiological mechanisms.

Two main types of trauma can cause this rupture: blunt trauma and penetrating trauma.

- **Blunt trauma:**

Blunt trauma has been described as the most common cause of aortic injury [27]. They are often caused by sudden deceleration [27], such as that encountered in high-speed vehicle accidents or falls from height.

In this type of impact, the aorta, which is firmly attached at several points along its course, undergoes intense stress when the body is suddenly braked, but the aorta attempts to keep moving due to inertia. This stress can lead to rupture of the aorta, often near the arterial ligament. In addition, patients with blunt trauma leading to aortic rupture often present with other severe thoracic injuries, such as multiple rib fractures or damage to intra-thoracic organs.

- **Penetrating trauma:**

In cases of penetrating trauma, such as gunshot wounds or stab wounds, damage to the aorta may result from direct injury to the aortic wall. The penetrating wound may cross the mediastinum, directly damaging the aorta.

2- Mechanisms of injury :

Traumatic rupture of the aorta can be caused by increased pressure, tensile or compressive forces, or a combination of these factors [1]. Hemodynamic factors, such as increased intra-thoracic pressure during trauma, and the mechanical mechanisms of thoracic deceleration and compression are crucial.

Ruptures, often due to shearing and stretching forces during abrupt deceleration [28], can also occur without direct thoracic impact, particularly at the aortic isthmus, a vulnerable zone in the event of tension between the fixed and mobile segments of the aorta.

Car accidents with sudden arrest of the thorax, falls from great heights, and side impacts increase the risk of such injuries [5, 28]. Although seatbelts reduce certain risks, they offer less protection against side impacts [29], which may result in rarer aortic injuries affecting the aortic arch or supra-sigmoid region.

Figure 1 summarizes the pathophysiological mechanisms of traumatic aortic injury.

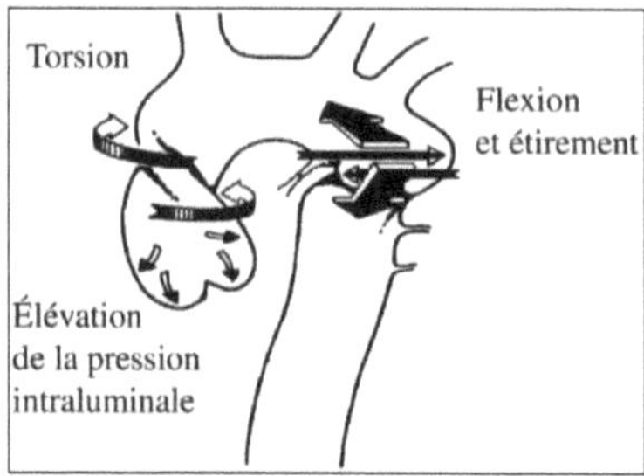

Figure 1: Pathophysiological mechanisms of traumatic aortic injury [30].

Studies on animal models, specifically swine [31], have shown that an initial tear in the intima and media of the aorta can occur under traumatic forces, leading to dissection. This may evolve into a pseudoaneurysm or complete rupture of the aorta. The time required for this to occur can vary, being influenced by factors such as increased blood pressure and afterload. In addition, interventions such as fluid resuscitation and rapid transfusions can accelerate this process.

Table III summarizes the main mechanisms involved in aortic trauma.

Table III: Main mechanisms involved in aortic trauma [32].

Mechanism	Description
Accelerationan d rapid deceleration	Significant deceleration occurs in frontal collisions and side impacts. The greatest risk is posed by front or side impacts.
Fall from a height d over 4 metres	High physical forces can cause blunt compression of the contents of the chest wall (in particular the aorta against the spine) and tearing of the aorta. This type of trauma can cause compression of the aorta in the region of the isthmus by the spine, sternum, first rib and collarbone.
Torsion against fastening points	Torsion of the aorta at the level of the arterial ligament just en can also lead to aortic trauma. can also lead to aortic trauma.
Injuries safety belt	Involves the abdominal aorta, although rarely injured in blunt trauma.
Other mechanisms high-risk	such as ejecting an unrestrained passenger from the vehicle and injuries resulting in death at the scene of the accident.

3- Anatomical lesions:

3- 1- Topography of traumatic aortic rupture :

The aorta is divided into five main segments, each with distinct anatomical and functional characteristics. These segments are the ascending aorta, the aortic arch, the descending thoracic portion, the supra-renal abdominal portion, and the sub-renal abdominal portion.

The aortic isthmus is a specific region of the aorta. Anatomically, it is located in the descending part of the thoracic aorta, just after the aortic arch. This area marks the transition between the aortic arch, which carries blood to the head and arms, and the descending thoracic aorta, which carries blood to the rest of the body. The aortic isthmus is clinically important, as it is often the site of lesions in

thoracic trauma, particularly in road accidents or falls from height.

This area is particularly vulnerable to injury due to its fixed position close to the spine and connection with the ligamentum arteriosus (the remnant of the ductus arteriosus), making it less mobile and more prone to shear forces during trauma. Consequently, the most frequent damage occurs at the aortic isthmus, downstream of the left subclavian artery [33, 34], and rarely above the aortic valves. If damaged, these valves can lead to immediately fatal traumatic aortic insufficiency by causing cardiac tamponade. In such cases, victims rarely survive long enough to be taken to a surgical center in time for treatment [35, 36]. According to the literature, 80 to 85% of victims die immediately from rupture in the pleural cavity and massive hemothorax [30, 35-37].

What's more, a third of patients with aortic isthmus rupture who arrive at hospital alive, die of secondary pleural rupture within the first twenty-four hours if left untreated [38, 39]. Only 5-10% of immediate survivors are still alive three months after the accident, often due to the development of a chronic aneurysm, which in turn can lead to secondary or late complications.

Involvement of other segments of the aorta is less frequent, including the proximal ascending aorta (8%-27%), the aortic arch (8%-18%) and the aorta. distal descending thoracic (11%-21%) [40]. However, among the 10-15% of casualties who initially survive the accident, the secondary mortality rate remains very high.

3- 2- Anatomical characteristics of aortic ruptures :

Ruptures of the thoracic aorta present a variety of anatomical characteristics, depending on their extent, either in thickness or width. In terms of thickness, there are two types of rupture:

-    **Complete ruptures:** These ruptures affect all three layers of the aorta (intima, media, adventitia). They are immediately fatal, unless the mediastinum and pleura can temporarily contain the bleeding.

-    **Incomplete breaks:** These breaks can be classified into two sub-categories:

-    Sub-adventitial: These are the most frequently observed clinical forms.

-    Isolated intimal: Difficult to diagnose, but unless serious.

In terms of width, the breaks are divided into :

-    **Circumferential ruptures:** here, retraction of the aorta's ends often results in a gap between the fragments and a misalignment of the aorta.

In the case of rupture at the isthmus, this can lead to verticalization of the aortic arch (Figure 2).

-    **Partial ruptures:** These ruptures affect only part of the circumference of the aorta, generally located in the concavity of the aorta, just after the arterial ligament.

It is important to note that the force required to cause an aortic tear is equivalent to an endovascular pressure of around 2500 mm Hg [24].

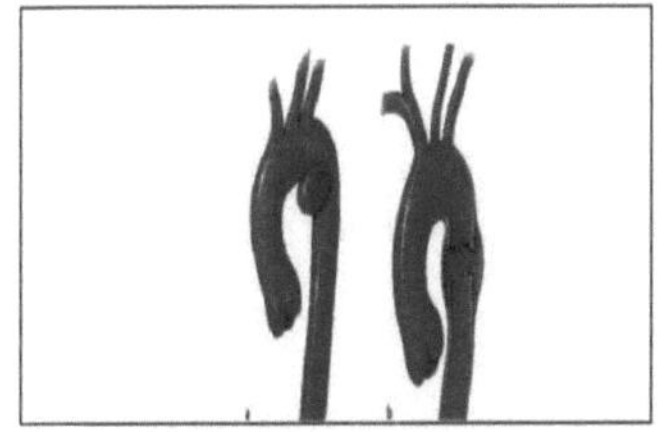

Figure 2: Circumferential extent of traumatic aortic rupture [24].

There is also a four-grade classification according to severity [24] (figure 3):

- Grade I: Intima tear.
- Grade II: Intramural hematoma.
- Grade III: Pseudoaneurysm.
- Grade IV: Complete aortic rupture.

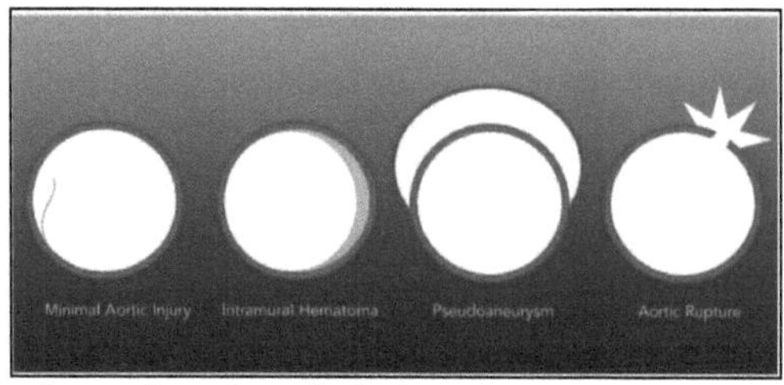

Figure 3: Grades of severity of aortic lesions [41].

3- 3- Anatomical and clinical evolution :

In the majority of cases, the natural course of traumatic rupture of the aortic isthmus tends towards complete rupture. This rupture may occur at different times. It is often immediate and sudden, resulting in death within a few hours.

minutes at the scene of the accident, or later, a few hours, days or weeks after the accident. It is sometimes triggered by minor physical effort, a coughing fit or a rise in blood pressure.

Four main evolutionary tables result from the nature of these ruptures [33, 42, 43]:

- **Immediate rupture of the three layers of aorta and pleura:** this leads to massive exsanguination, and survival is very short.

- **Acute fissured hemomediastinum:** In this situation, the mediastinal hematoma, filtering through the pleura, partially covers the breach thanks to the distended adventitia, resulting in slow, continuous hemorrhage. This lesion can lead to immediate or delayed hemothorax, evolving rapidly within 24 hours, and causing early mortality.

- **Hemo-mediastinum due to secondary rupture of a false aneurysm:** A false aneurysm forms, held in place by the adventitia and pleura, allowing blood flow to continue, but with the risk of secondary rupture after a latency period of several days to a few weeks.

- **Organized hematoma:** In this rarer case, the aneurysmal pocket consolidates through fibrosis, and may even calcify, forming a chronic aneurysm discovered months or years after the event [43].

The prognosis of traumatic aortic rupture (TAT) is influenced by the location of the rupture and the severity of damage to the aortic wall. Complete ruptures, involving all layers of the aorta, may not be fatal before surgery, thanks to the mediastinal hematoma and visceral pleura that restrict blood flow. Aortic tears are generally transverse and linear, but longitudinal fissures can occur. Ruptures may be partial

or complete, with an increased risk of secondary rupture in the case of complete separation. Intimal lesions, which are difficult to diagnose, may heal spontaneously or evolve into a false aneurysm, with an uncertain prognosis.

3.4. Associated lesions :

In cases of traumatic rupture of the aorta, it is common to find associated lesions, especially in cases of severe trauma. These additional lesions can complicate diagnosis, pose problems in prioritizing surgical interventions, and severely affect prognosis. Studies have shown a close correlation between mortality and the severity of these associated lesions [1].

Traumatic injuries to the thoracic aorta are often accompanied by multiple other lesions [44, 45]. Non-survivors have an average of four associated injuries, while survivors have two [46]. Craniocerebral, facial, pulmonary, cardiac, abdominal and bone injuries are among the most frequent [47]. Bone injuries, including vertebral and limb fractures, are also common and may become a priority emergency, complicating the management of aortic rupture [5]. Thus, it is crucial to systematically investigate these associated lesions with a rapid but comprehensive workup, using standard radiographs, abdominal ultrasound and full-body CT scans.

V- Diagnosis of traumatic rupture of the aorta: 1- Diagnosis of severity:

Multiple lesions frequently coexist in aortic trauma [48]. The reception and management of polytraumatized patients with suspected traumatic injury to the aorta in the emergency department are key moments in the history of aortic trauma.

These are critical conditions that require a comprehensive and systematic clinical assessment right from the pre-hospital phase. On arrival in the emergency department, from triage onwards and throughout the entire course of care, the management of casualties is guided by a rigorous, structured approach, often represented by the acronym ABCDE [49]. It includes a respiratory, hemodynamic and neurological examination, as well as the taking of vital vitals. The aim of this assessment is to rapidly identify any obvious or potential distress requiring immediate intervention.

1-1- Respiratory distress :

The upper airways must be checked for freedom, and secured if at risk. Everything must be done while respecting the straightness of the head-neck-torso axis, and mobilizing the cervical spine as soon as there is clinical suspicion of cervical damage, or in the presence of severe head trauma.

Signs of respiratory distress such as respiratory rate (RR) > 25 cycles/min, cyanosis, signs of respiratory struggle, or oxygen desaturation < 90% should be detected. Pulmonary auscultation may be normal or reveal a unilateral decrease in breath sounds.

1- 2- Circulatory distress :

It is essential to look for PAS < 90 mm Hg accompanied by tachycardia (HR > 120 beats/min). These symptoms may be associated with signs of peripheral hypotension such as mottling, cold extremities and cold sweats. Chest pain should also be sought. In cases of acute aortic dissection, collapse and shock are frequent presentations. The hemorrhagic origin of shock is often suspected, and management follows the principles of permissive hypotensive resuscitation, with the hemodynamic aim of obtaining a perceptible radial pulse.

If shock is cardiogenic in origin, pathologies such as aortic insufficiency and coronary artery disease are often involved, necessitating the use of positive inotropes. If cardiac tamponade is detected by trans-thoracic echocardiography (TTE) at the patient's bedside, urgent surgical intervention is required.

These findings underscore the importance of careful clinical assessment and early intervention for thoracic trauma patients, to prevent complications and optimize outcomes.

Systematic analysis of the electrocardiogram (ECG) is crucial for detecting signs of myocardial ischemia or pericardial effusion, ashighlighted by various studies. Rathachai Kaewlai et al [50] highlighted a higher rate of blunt cardiac lesions in patients with thoracic aortic lesions, compared with those without, emphasizing the importance of the ECG in diagnosing such lesions.

In addition, the study by Mucahit Emet et al [51] revealed low sensitivity and specificity of the ECG when used in isolation shortly after trauma. Kimberly Nagy et al [52] concluded that there was no need for further intervention in patients with blunt chest trauma, a normal ECG, normal blood pressure and no rhythm disturbances on admission.

1- 3- Neurological distress:

Neurological deficits, such as hemiplegic, monoplegic, aphasic or sensory symptoms, may be related to an interruption of blood flow in a carotid artery. In the absence of associated cranial or cervical trauma, these symptoms are of particular concern. The occurrence of syncope should raise the suspicion of cardiac tamponade or supra-aortic trunk dissection [53].

In summary, the initial clinical assessment in the emergency department of polytraumatized patients with possible traumatic injury to the aorta is a complex and detailed process, requiring careful attention at every stage of the examination to detect and effectively manage the various forms of vital distress.

2- Clinical features suggestive of the diagnosis of acute traumatic rupture of the aorta :

Acute traumatic rupture of the aorta in the context of polytrauma is often obscured by other injuries, making its diagnosis complex. It is crucial to suspect this condition in specific accidents such as high-speed road collisions, falls from great heights, or severe crush injuries.

2- 1- Interrogatory :

Any trauma should arouse suspicion of aortic rupture, especially if the circumstances of the accident suggest it. When questioning the patient, it is important to ascertain whether the mechanism of the accident was :

- A traffic accident involving sudden deceleration, ejection or a high-speed collision (car, motorcycle), with the potential for fatalities among the other victims.

- A fall from a great height, such as defenestration, an aerial sports accident (skydiving, hang-gliding, flying) or work at height (scaffolding, elevator).

- Crushing under a heavy load, as in an elevator accident or earthquake.

- It is also important to look for signs of paraplegia or paraparesis, even if transient, immediately after the accident, as these are often indicative of aortic injury. These neurological symptoms may result from temporary or permanent, partial or complete impairment of blood flow to the spinal cord, directly attributable to the aortic injury.

2- 2- Physical examination :

The physical examination must be meticulous from head to toe. It should look for :

Respiratory compromise: may be caused by a variety of mechanisms, including acute pulmonary edema linked to heart failure, myocardial ischemia, or large-scale hemothorax due to bleeding in the pleura. These situations can result in cataclysmic hemorrhage, rapidly leading to death if not treated urgently.

- Auscultation to detect a diastolic murmur indicating aortic insufficiency.
- Pericardial friction: may indicate irritation or inflammation of the pericardium, often due to effusion or bleeding in the pericardial cavity.
- Jugular turgor: another important sign, indicating increased venous pressure, potentially due to right heart failure or tamponade.
- Peripheral pulse asymmetry.
- Measurement of blood pressure in all 4 limbs is essential to detect any significant disparity. In fact, all road accident victims should have their blood pressure measured in all four limbs [1].

Regarding post-traumatic aortic hypertension, historical studies such as those by La Foret in 1965 [54], highlighted its diagnostic role, considering it to be a result of acute coarctation due to hematoma. However, later research challenged this theory, finding no significant difference in pressure between the upper and lower limbs. More recent hypotheses [55] suggest that hypertension may be due to stimulation of sympathetic nerve fibers in the aortic isthmus, triggering reflex hypertension.

Blood pressure and pulse asymmetry may indicate a rupture or dissection of the aorta, leading to differential perfusion of the upper limbs. This is a crucial finding for emergency physicians, as it can rapidly lead to a diagnosis of aortic injury [56].

Minor neurological deficits: may occur due to the impact of the trauma on the central or peripheral nervous system, or as a consequence of hypo-perfusion due to hemodynamic instability.

- Acute limb ischemia: may be the result of vascular obstruction caused by aortic dissection or thrombus following associated arterial trauma.

- Hemodynamic instability and syncope: may indicate severe acute hypotension, often due to a large aortic lesion, and require immediate assessment and intervention to prevent a fatal outcome.

- The hoarseness of the voice, often following injury to the laryngeal recurrent nerve, is another potential clue, especially if the aortic trauma is close to the aortic arch [56].

These elements are essential for a rapid and accurate diagnosis in an emergency situation, guiding towards an aortic lesion requiring immediate intervention.

2- 3- Complementary examinations :

- **The FAST examination (Focused Assessment with Sonography for Trauma:**

It is a simple, safe, sensitive, non-invasive and reproducible procedure, commonly performed in emergency departments. It is imperative to perform it in all severely traumatized patients, as it can show indirect signs of traumatic aortic rupture, such as tamponade (Figure 4), major pleural effusion or intraperitoneal effusion [57, 58].

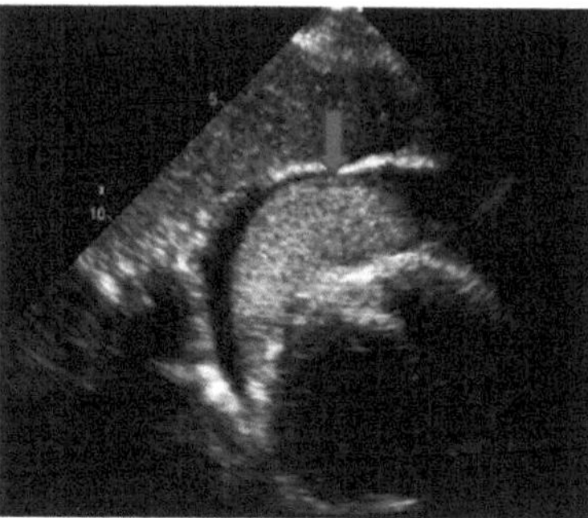

Figure 4: Cardiac tamponade caused by a large pericardial hematoma (red arrow) revealed by FAST echo [59].

- **Standard chest X-ray:**

A frontal chest X-ray is often the first radiological examination performed at the patient's bedside to suggest a traumatic rupture of the aorta [60]. It may show the presence of a mediastinal hematoma [61]. Classical signs include enlargement of the mediastinum. This is suspected when the

width of the mediastinum/thorax width at the aortic arch exceeds 0.25, or when the width of the mediastinum at this level exceeds 8 cm (figure 5).

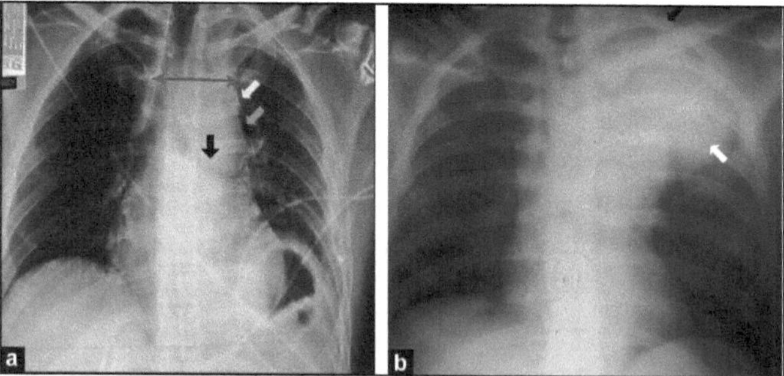

Figure 5: Radiographic image of a ruptured aortic isthmus with signs to look for: a: anteroposterior projection: widening of the mediastinum : double red arrow), disappearance of the contours of the aortic button (yellow arrow), lowering of the left main bronchus (black arrow), opacification of the space between the aorta and the pulmonary artery (green arrow); b: anteroposterior projection: left hemothorax (white arrow), apical cap (black arrow) [62].

Although mediastinal enlargement is a significant sign, it is not specific to this pathology, and its diagnostic value may vary depending on several factors, including the radiographic techniques employed.

It is important to note that only 20% of mediastinal hematomas result from closed aortic lesions [61]. This enlargement may also arise from other types of injury, such as damage to the large mediastinal vessels, or injury to the small vessels following fractures of the sternum, clavicle, ribs or vertebrae [63, 64].

Mediastinal width measurements may be distorted by factors such as vascular engorgement in trauma patients or conditions such as aortic ectasia, mediastinal lipomatosis or lymphadenopathy [63-65].

On frontal chest X-rays, a hemomediastinum resulting from an aortic lesion at the aortic isthmus may also obscure the aorto-pulmonary window, shift the trachea to the right, and lower or deflect the left main bronchus and esophagus, as identified by a radiopaque nasogastric tube [64, 66].

Various radiological signs are associated with closed traumatic aortic injury, such as widening, blurring or irregularity of the aortic button, widening of the paravertebral shadows or a hemi-thorax, mainly on the left side in 90% of cases.

Table IV shows the relevance of the various radiological signs for the diagnosis of traumatic aortic lesions in terms of sensitivity and specificity according to the literature [61].

Table IV: Radiological signs for the diagnosis of traumatic aortic lesions: Sensitivity and specificity [61].

Caractéristiques	Sensibilité (%)	Spécificité (%)
Directement liées à la lésion aortique :		
Irrégularité ou flou du contour du bouton aortique	72	47
Élargissement du bouton aortique	35	60
Liées à la présence d'un hématome médiastinal		
Élargissement médiastinal	90	19
Opacification de la fenêtre aorto-pulmonaire	42	83
Déplacement de la paroi latérale gauche de l'œsophage ou d'un tube naso-gastrique	9	96
Déplacement de la paroi latérale gauche de la trachée ou d'un tube endotrachéal	20	92
Trachée antérieure déplacée sur les vues latérales	ND	ND
Déplacement vers le bas de la bronche souche gauche	3	99
Silhouette cardiaque élargie et perte de définition	7	96
Déplacement vers la droite de la veine cave supérieure	ND	ND
Obscurcissement des veines azygos	ND	ND
Autres caractéristiques :		
Chapeau extrapleural apical gauche	5	96
Opacification de la bordure médiale du poumon gauche	12	95
Hémothorax gauche	15	97
Épaississement de la bande para-vertébrale droite ou gauche	30	99
Épaississement de la bande para-sternale droite ou gauche	2	97
ND : Non Disponible		

- **Computed tomography or multi-slice CT :**

Multi-bar spiral CT is the Gold Standard for emergency diagnosis of traumatic aortic rupture. It is used to detect aortic lesions following trauma, indicated by clinical or radiological clues. If a lesion is confirmed by this scan, the patient is referred to a cardiovascular surgeon. A normal result excludes the presence of aortic lesions.

Thoracic aortography is reserved for cases where aortographic spiral CT reveals hemomediastinum without features of aortic lesion, which concerns less than 5% of patients [61].

Two-dimensional and three-dimensional reconstructions provide valuable anatomical information for the cardiovascular surgeon. The American College of Radiology recommends non-contrast CT, followed by CT angiography, as initial imaging methods for traumatic aortic lesions [67].

The scanner is fast and reliable, detecting not only aortic ruptures, but also other possible lesions caused by the violence of the trauma.

Cerebral, cervical, thoracic and abdominal lesions can be initially detected by FAST ultrasound and confirmed by CT scan. Since its introduction, CT has evolved, with helical acquisition revolutionizing vascular imaging with 100% sensitivity, 96% specificity and 100% negative predictive value, essential for accurate assessment prior to endovascular treatment [12].

CT scanning, used to detect traumatic aortic lesions, comprises two phases: the first without injection to look for high-density infiltration of periaortic fat, and the second with injection to identify signs of aortic injury such as increased aortic caliber, irregularities in vascular contour, parietal notches or intimal flaps.

These examinations are superior to angiography for detecting isolated lesions of the inner tunica of the aorta, and monitoring their evolution without surgical repair [1].

Radiological features of traumatic aortic lesions include direct (aortic wall alterations) and indirect (periaortic mediastinal hematoma, pleural effusions, hemothorax) signs, crucial for planning procedures such as endovascular stent insertion.

Signs of aortic injury sought include [34, 61, 68, 69]:

- Curvilinear intimal flaring: This means that the inner wall of the aorta is deformed in the shape of a curve.

- Intramural hematoma or dissection: Intramural hematoma is defined as an accumulation of blood inside the wall of the aorta, often due to an internal tear. Aortic dissection occurs when the layers of the aortic wall separate due to blood pressure, creating a space for blood to seep through.

- Irregularities of the aortic wall or contour.

- Pseudoaneurysm: a protrusion in the aortic wall that forms as a result of injury and may be filled with blood.

- Pseudo-coarctation: This means that there is an apparent constriction or narrowing of the aorta.

- Hemomediastinum: This is an indirect sign of aortic injury, as bleeding may originate from the aorta or other vascular structures.

- Mediastinal hematoma (soft tissue infiltration).

- Location of hemomediastinum: The location of the hemomediastinum may have diagnostic significance. For example, if the bleeding surrounds the aorta and other vascular structures, this is more suggestive of a vascular lesion.

These signs are essential for the diagnosis and evaluation of traumatic aortic lesions.

The quality of the CT examination may be influenced by various factors (inability to raise the arms, patient agitation, inability to hold the arms, etc.).

apnea), and in these cases, if the diagnosis is unclear, angiography remains a necessary option.

Table V summarizes the scanographic grades of traumatic aortic injury.

Table V: Classification of thoracic aortic lesions proposed by Starnes et al, based on angioscan imaging features[34, 70]:

Catégories	Caractéristiques	Exemples
Grade 1 : Lacération intimale (Flèche jaune)	-Aucun changement externe du contour de l'aorte. -Petite déchirure avec moins de 10 mm de thrombus. -Peut être parfois traité de manière conservatrice.	
Grade 2 : Grand flap intimal (Flèche jaune)	-Aucun changement externe du contour de l'aorte. -Thrombus visible de plus de 10 mm.	
Grade 3 : Pseudo-anévrisme (Flèche jaune)	-Aspect bulbeux avec changement du contour de l'aorte. -Rupture contenue.	
Grade 4 : Rupture (Flèche jaune)	-Le patient est rarement suffisamment stable pour une imagerie. -Du produit de contraste extravasé au-delà du contour aortique	

- **Transthoracic ultrasonography (TTE):**

Despite its limitations, transthoracic ultrasound is crucial for the initial diagnosis of aortic lesions and their complications, thanks to its immediate availability, particularly in unstable patients. It is less reliable for direct assessment dlesions of the thoracic aorta, but helps to detect the severity of aortic insufficiency and to measure pericardial effusion warranting rigorous monitoring.

However, trans-thoracic echocardiography is often suboptimal [61], particularly in the evaluation of severe chest trauma, in the presence of conditions such as chest wall hematomas, subcutaneous emphysema, pneumothorax, pulmonary contusion and/or mediastinal emphysema. It can sometimes detect a flap in the proximal part of the ascending thoracic aorta, but its limitations in visualizing specific anatomical details must be taken into account.

- **Transesophageal echocardiography (TEE):**

It plays a crucial role in the diagnosis of aortic lesions, particularly in the context of mediastinal hematomas, although its performance is inferior to that of CT or angiography in terms of sensitivity and specificity [24,46]. Ideal for mechanically ventilated patients, TEE can be performed rapidly and without specific precautions as soon as polytrauma patients arrive at hospital. In non-intubated patients, it is crucial to exclude a cervical spine fracture before proceeding with the examination.

Thanks to its positioning in the immediate vicinity of the aortic isthmus, TEE offers detailed and comprehensive visualization of this region [71], providing two-dimensional images and high-resolution color Doppler data.

This technology is particularly effective in distinguishing different forms of aortic lesions, such as subadventitial ruptures and traumatic aortic dissections

[71,72], characterized by signs such as intimal flaps, aortic wall hematomas, pseudoaneurysms, aortic occlusions and deformations of the circular shape of the descending aorta.

Here are the various ultrasound signs observed in traumatic rupture of the aorta:

-       Fusiform dilatation of the descending aorta.

-       Saccular aneurysm with neck of descending aorta (Figure 6).

-       Alteration of the circular shape of the descending aorta.

-       Wall flaps of varying thickness are present in the aorta, indicating laceration of the parietal tunics (Figure 7).

-       Thrombus in the aorta, either mural or pedicled and mobile (Figure 8).

-       Aortic occlusions, linked to pseudocoarctation syndrome.

-       Hemomediastinum, confirmed by TEE, crucial for determining whether the aortic wall lesion is trans-mural.

However, TEE has certain limitations and contraindications. It is inadvisable in non-intubated patients with cervical spine fractures, and may vary in quality depending on the expertise of the operator. What's more, it fails to explore the entire circumference of the aorta in around 30% of cases, particularly in the presence of significant mediastinal hematoma.

In parallel, intravascular ultrasound complements TEE by providing real-time, high-resolution transverse axial images of the aorta. This tool is useful for

to clarify subtle aortic anomalies undetectable by thoracic aortography, but is limited by the high cost of probes [61] and sometimes incomplete visualization of the aorta in tortuous or ulcerated regions.

In conclusion, although TEE is a safe, accurate and rapid method fr assessing thoracic trauma and suspected aortic dissection, its limitations and contraindications must be taken into account.

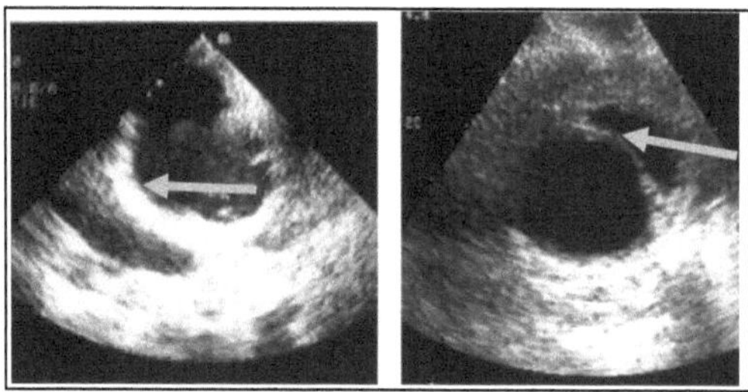

Figure 6: Various presentations of traumatic false aneurysms at the aortic isthmus seen on transesophageal ultrasound indicated by yellow arrow [33].

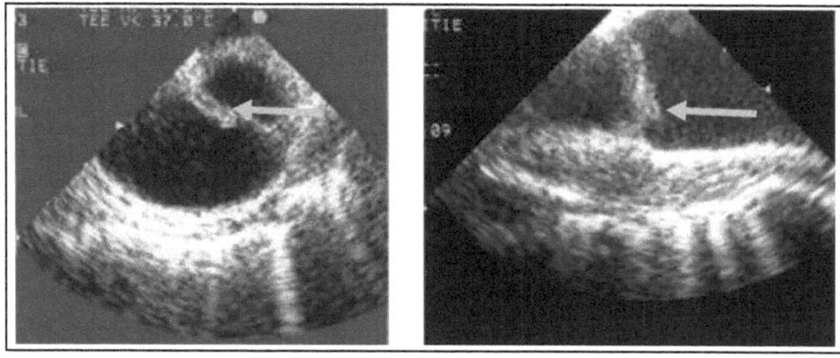

Figure 7: Transesophageal echocardiography identifies a medial flap, indicated by a yellow arrow, revealing a laceration of the aortic wall, with visualization of the injury in 0-degree transverse and longitudinal sections [33].

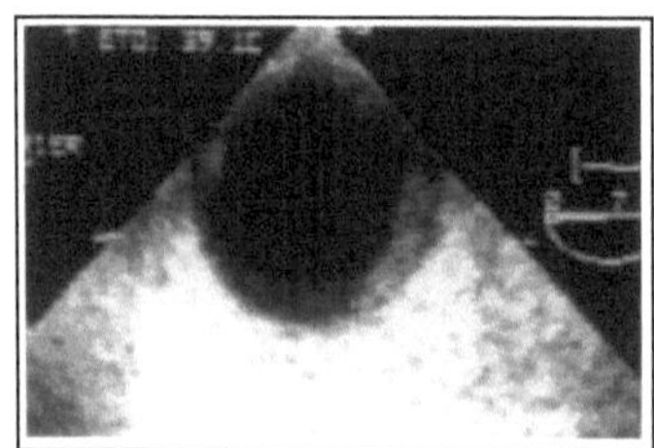

Figure 8: Transesophageal echocardiographic presentation of an intramural hematoma in the descending thoracic aorta following trauma, indicated by a yellow arrow [33].

- **Aortography:**

Thoracic aortography plays a crucial role in detecting, localizing and determining the extent of aortic lesions, as well as defining the anatomy of the branches of the aortic arch. It stands out for its high sensitivity (96%) and specificity (98%) in detecting these injuries [61, 63, 65, 73].

False positives or negatives may result from incomplete image series or inadequate injections, or may be confused with ductal diverticula or ulcerated atheromas [63, 73, 74].

Historically, aortography was the gold standard for the diagnosis of traumatic aortic lesions [61], but it has been superseded by CT, which is more sensitive and specific.

It is now limited to certain specific cases, such as the insertion of endovascular stents (Figure 9), after embolization in cases of hemorrhagic shock and suspected traumatic rupture of the aortic isthmus (TTIR) in patients with lateralized signs of aortic injury, but no definitive lesion identified on CT scan [34].

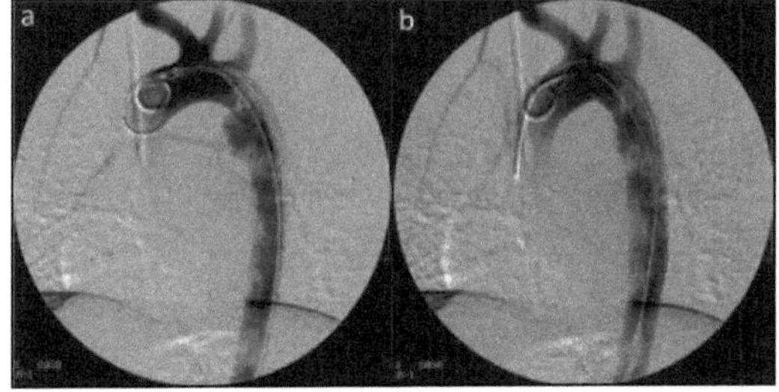

Figure 9: Angiographic image showing a pseudoaneurysm at the aortic isthmus, indicated by an arrow (a), followed by deployment of a 21 mm Gore thoracic aortic stent (b) via a right femoral approach,enabling immediate exclusion of the pseudoaneurysm [34].

2- 4- Diagnostic approach in the emergency department :

To identify traumatic aortic injury in severely injured patients, particularly those who have experienced significant deceleration or whose chest X-ray reveals possible AVR, aortic angioscan or TEE is recommended [75]. Both methods are equally sensitive and specific [76]. Their use depends essentially on the patient's clinical condition and the specific assessments required.

For patients with hemodynamic instability, TEE is preferred, as it enables direct bedside hemodynamic assessment (including evaluation of blood volume and cardiac function), as well as diagnosis of aortic injury. On the other hand, CT scanning, which has become a fundamental element in the comprehensive assessment of polytrauma patients, is frequently used because it is more widely available than TEE.

The assessment and management of traumatic lesions of the aorta are crucial due to their potential for rapid aggravation. According to the medical literature [77],several clinical signs may indicate a worsening of the aortic lesion, and justify a follow-up thoracic CT scan prior to stenting.

These signs include:

- Aggravated or new chest pain

- Hypotension or signs of shock indicating internal bleeding or cardiovascular deterioration

- Heart rhythm disorders

- Breathing difficulties or hypoxia

- A change in peripheral pulses

- Neurological signs such as confusion or paralysis.

The decision to carry out a thoracic CT scan must take into account the overall clinical picture. Each case is unique and requires individual assessment.

VI- Therapeutic management :

The initial management of patients with traumatic rupture of the aorta is crucial and must be carried out in accordance with best practice recommendations, with a multidisciplinary approach involving an emergency physician, an anesthesiologist-intensive care physician, a radiologist, a cardiovascular surgeon and a cardiologist. This collaboration aims to improve prognosis by intervening as early as the pre-hospital phase. Key objectives include :

- Stabilizing vital distress
- Primary assessment via FAST echo ± chest X-ray in bed,
- Complete lesion assessment by whole-body CT scan
- Prioritizing care for various injuries
- Performing emergency hemostasis
- And referring the patient to the most appropriate structure for further care.
- This approach is based on both general and specific measures.

1-   General measures :

Initial resuscitation measures and provisional injury assessment are carried out on site by the EMS team, or on arrival in the dehospitalization room.

Initial treatment of polytrauma in trauma centers follows advanced trauma life support protocols.

However, for patients with ATN, particular attention should be paid to blood pressure and heart rate because of their effects on wound extension and rupture [40].

One or more obvious or potential life-threatening conditions must be sought and treated according to the ABCDE approach, bearing in mind the possibility of vertebral damage.

Treatment of traumatic injuries is prioritized according to their immediate vital risk. Major haemorrhages and intracranial injuries with mass effect are given priority [78].

In the event of hemodynamic instability, all measures are taken to maintain a satisfactory respiratory and hemodynamic state, including intubation, mechanical ventilation, vascular filling, transfusions, administration of catecholamines, surgical hemostasis, or embolization.

The ABCDE approach is preferred for organizing this management [78,79]. The frequent presentations of collapse and shock, often associated with hypotension (PAS<90 mm Hg) and tachycardia (HR>120 beats/min), are mainly due to a hemorrhagic origin, and resuscitation follows the permissive hypotension algorithm. In the event of tamponade, pericardial drainage is indicated.

Permissive hypotension may not be tolerated in cases of other concomitant injuries, where adequate organ perfusion requires higher arterial pressures [40].

For hemodynamically stable patients without catecholamines, recommended antihypertensive therapies include esmolol, labetalol, clivedipine, nicardipine, urapidil, and clonidine, administered intravenously to maintain systolic blood pressure below 120 mm Hg, diastolic blood pressure below 100 mm Hg, and heart rate between 60 and 80 bpm [80].

Targets may be adjusted according to the perfusion status of other organs and surgical urgency. In the absence of contraindications, short-acting β-blockers are preferred; otherwise, non-dihydropyridine calcium channel blockers are used, aiming for an anti-impulsive effect to reduce aortic wall stress [81].

2-   Specific care :

2- 1- Preoperative assessment :

Implantation of aortic stents or open surgery for traumatic aortic lesions requires rigorous preoperative evaluation, including angioscan to specify the anatomy and select the appropriate prosthesis, minimizing the risk of endoleaks [82]. A complete blood work-up is essential, assessing haemostasis, renal and liver function, and CPK and troponin levels, to anticipate complications and adjust post-operative management. These steps are vital to the success of the operation and the reduction of complications.

2- 2- Processing time :

Optimal management of traumatic aortic lesions, particularly with regard to the timing of surgery, has evolved over the years, thanks to a variety of studies and technological advances.

Initially, surgical intervention in extreme emergency was advocated, following the work of Parmley [44]. However, as early as the 1970s, this approach was challenged by Akins [83], who advocated delayed treatment of aortic lesions, particularly in patients with major associated lesions. Today, it is recognized that there is a benefit to delayed management of contained isthmus rupture, especially in patients with a severe lesion work-up [84], provided that blood pressure control is optimal [15].

Recent studies have confirmed this attitude. Indeed, some studies [85] have shown that delayed management of traumatic aortic lesions is associated with good short- and long-term results, with no significant difference between surgical and endovascular repair.

Other studies [86] have also shown that patients operated on after 24 hours have better survival than those operated on within the first 24 hours, despite similar injury patterns. Research [87] has revealed that the probability of secondary aortic rupture is around 4%, varying between 2% and 5% according to different studies. This rate is lower than that of associated mortality.

to the early use of heparin or extracorporeal circulation (ECC) in the treatment of hemorrhagic lung and brain injuries, estimated at between 3% and 33% [24].

With the advent of endovascular treatment (EVT), it has become increasingly indicated due to the absence of complications associated with CEC and the intensive use of heparin, necessary in conventional surgical procedures [88].

In summary, the ideal timing for surgery of traumatic aortic lesions depends on the severity of associated injuries, patient stability, and technical resources. Advances in endovascular techniques offer less invasive options, suitable even for complex cases, enabling deferred intervention if necessary.

2- 3. surgical treatment :

The management of ATN has historically relied on emergency surgery as soon as the diagnosis is made, aimed at reducing the risk of death from aortic rupture [12].

However, this urgent surgical approach has a high mortality rate, of around 30% according to studies [12,47]. Factors increasing the risk of mortality include the patient's advanced age, pre-existing cardiovascular and respiratory conditions, and the presence of bleeding [47].

Moreover, surgery often requires extracorporeal circulation and early heparinization [12], which can exacerbate other lesions, notably cerebral, pulmonary or abdominal [89].

In some studies, all deaths occurred within 48 hours of surgery [12]. Conventional surgery is still indicated for young, stable patients [90], at low risk of bleeding, and when surgery can be postponed by a few hours.

The factors that may influence the choice between open surgery and an endovascular approach for the treatment of traumatic aortic injury depend on several clinical considerations[90] :

- Anatomy of the aorta: Anatomical anomalies such as severe curvature or calcification of the aorta can make endovascular access difficult or impossible.
- Other lesions or medical conditions: The presence of other traumatic

lesions, particularly those affecting areas where the endovascular material would be positioned or those that could be aggravated by an endovascular procedure, may favor open surgery.

-    General state of health: Underlying conditions such as severe vascular disease or coagulation abnormalities may influence the choice of procedure.

-    Availabilitý and expertise: the availabilitý of endovascular material and the expertise of the surgical team can also be determining factors.

-    Patient preferences and consent: Patient preferences, based on information provided on the risks and benefits of each approach, also play an important role in the decision.

2- 4- Thoracic endovascular aortic repair :

The introduction of the first endovascular thoracic stent graft by Volodos et al. in 1991 marked a revolution in the treatment of AVR, paving the way for less invasive management that was better suited to high-risk patients and victims of polytrauma [88]. Subsequent studies have attested to the efficacy of endovascular treatment, highlighting its positive impact on prognosis and offering it as a promising solution for aortic emergencies, validated by satisfactory short- and medium-term results [91,92].

Currently, TEV has become the preferred strategy for treating RTA, particularly in polytraumatized patients, thanks to its many advantages over traditional surgery [93]. The technique stands out for its ability to be undertaken immediately, regardless of other lesions present, due to its minimally invasive nature. It requires only limited vascular access in an uninjured area, avoiding aortic clamping and the need for significant anticoagulation, or even no anticoagulation at all in the case of associated hemorrhage [88].

The minimally invasive nature of the endovascular procedure makes it the alternative of choice, particularly in cases where open surgery would present greater risks. It can be performed without excessive patient mobilization, heparinization or aortic clamping. The benefits of endovascular stenting extend beyond the avoidance of left thoracotomy, single-pulmonary ventilation and systemic anticoagulation, which is crucial in patients with severe trauma.

The rapidity and simplicity of this technique reduce the patient's exposure to operative risks, and enable it to be applied simultaneously to the management of other priority lesions during the same operative time. This relatively safe procedure is also suitable for older patients with other concomitant pathologies.

VTE is associated with a lower risk of paraplegia compared with conventional surgical methods.

However, TEV has technical limitations [94], notably small diameters of the thoracic aorta or pronounced curvatures of the aortic arch.

When the femoral arteries prove too narrow, it may be necessary to opt for primary iliac or even direct aortic access. It's worth mentioning that coverage of the left subclavian artery by the stent graft is achieved in around a quarter of cases, with no signs of limb ischemia.

Finally, leaks around the stent, known as endoleaks, although relatively rare, occur in 5.3% of cases post-operatively [12]. These complications are of particular concern in the long-term follow-up of VTE patients.

2- 5- Choice of treatment strategy :

2- 5- 1- Approach to the initial management of traumatic aortic injury:

As part of our analysis, we incorporated the recommendations of the 2022 ACC/AHA Guidelines for the Diagnosis and Management of Aortic Disease, which provide a guiding framework for clinicians in the treatment of AVR [40].

Decision-making in the management of acute traumatic injuries of the aorta due bblunt trauma requires a careful approach, given the complexity and dynamics of the factors involved.

This complexity is particularly evident when considering the different management strategies for different grades of ALR, ranging from a non-operative approach to more invasive surgical interventions.

- *RTA grade 1 :*

Grade 1 aortic lesions are considered to have a high probability of spontaneous resolution and are associated with an extremely low risk of aortic-related death.

Management of these cases generally involves a conservative medical approach, with careful follow-up imaging to confirm resolution of the injury. This approach is supported by previous research, such as that conducted by Estrera [10], which found that medical management of Grade 1 injuries resulted in a 0% mortality rate.

Accordingly, current Society for Vascular Surgery (SVS) guidelines recommend expectant management for grade 1 injuries, with surgical repair considered only for higher-grade injuries.

- *RTA grade 2 :*

The data indicate that injury grade is an independent predictor of aorta-related death. However, the results for grade 1 and 2 injuries appear similar, whether treatment is non-operative or by endovascular technique. This observation is consistent, including for in-hospital and aorta-related death rates. One high-volume center even reported no significant difference in mortality rates between non-operative and operative strategies for grade 1 and 2 injuries [95].

For patients presenting a grade 2 lesion with high-risk imaging features, aortic intervention is deemed reasonable. These high-risk features include elements such as a posterior mediastinal hematoma of

more than 10 mm, a lesion size to aortic diameter ratio greater than 1.4, or a mediastinal hematoma causing a mass effect.

On the other hand, for Grade 2 patients without these high-risk features, non-operative management with follow-up imaging could be envisaged.

- ***RTA grades 3 and 4:***

Grade 3 and 4 injuries present a high risk of progression and rupture, thus requiring urgent intervention. In the case of grade 3 injuries, non-operative treatment has been identified as an independent predictor of all-cause mortality, underlining the importance of prompt intervention in these cases [96].

In summary, the management of ATN varies considerably depending on the grade of injury and the specific characteristics of each case. A thorough, individualized assessment is crucial to determine the most appropriate management strategy for each patient, taking into account the potential risks and benefits of different approaches.

2- 5- 2- Endovascular repair versus open surgery :

Endovascular treatment has gradually come to be regarded as the approach of choice for traumatic lesions of the thoracic aorta. This is corroborated by trends observed between 2007 and 2015, during which time there was a significant decrease in open thoracic aortic repairs, from 7.5% to 1.9%. At the same time, the adoption of endovascular repair increased significantly, climbing from 12.1% to 25.7%.

Despite the absence of randomized trials directly comparing open repair with endovascular management [97], a synthesis of data from trauma registries and meta-analyses reveals significant benefits associated with VTE in patients with compatible anatomy. These benefits include improved short-term mortality rates, as well as a reduction in ischemic spinal cord complications and cases of acute kidney injury.

However, when treating polytrauma patients, peri-operative heparin management, which is necessary to prevent thrombo-embolic complications during VTE, may increase the increased risk of bleeding. A careful assessment of overall bleeding risk is therefore essential for each patient prior to heparin administration. A small study of VTE, mainly in patients with Grade 3 AVR, showed no significant differences in bleeding, thrombo-embolic complications or mortality, whether full-dose, low-dose or no heparin was used. It should be noted, however, that patients who received a full dose of heparin underwent repair 3 times longer than those who did not [98].

In terms of specific support for the recommendation, some studies have shown that compared with open repair, endovascular treatment of AVR results in improved procedural and 30-day mortality rates, and also contributes to a reduction in post-operative complications, including spinal cord injury and acute kidney injury [11, 99]. A meta-analysis of 17 retrospective studies associated VTE with lower procedural and 30-day mortality rates, as well as a significant reduction in cases of post-operative paraplegia [11]. Similar conclusions were drawn by Murad et al [100], who,

after analyzing 139 studies involving 7768 patients, reported marked reductions in mortality and ICS. Data from the National Trauma Data Bank, which aggregates multi-centric information from trauma centers, confirm these findings, describing reduced mortality, shorter ICU and hospital stays, as well as lower rates of acute kidney injury and acute respiratory distress syndrome for patients treated with VTE compared with those who underwent open repair [99].

Despite the advantages of endovascular repair, open surgery remains relevant in cases where endovascular techniques are not applicable or prove inadequate, particularly in children and small patients [101, 102], or when endovascular options are unsuitable.

The option of open surgery is considered according to various determining factors, which are:

- The location and nature of the lesion: Open surgery is often preferred when the lesion is located in areas of the aorta where stent placement is technically impractical. Lesions close to vital structures, such as the aortic arch where major branches emerge, may make stent implantation difficult, and thus favor open repair.

- Size and extent of lesion: When faced with long or complex lesions, the endovascular approach may prove insufficient to provide a stable and safe repair. In such cases, the option of open surgery may offer a more suitable and durable solution [103].

- Patient's condition: Some patients may have specific contraindications to the use of stents, such as allergies to materials.

or anatomical features that compromise stent placement or function.

For these individuals, open surgery may represent the only viable alternative.

- Failure of minimally invasive approaches: In some cases, previous attempts at endovascular repair have failed or led to complications. In these situations, open surgery may become necessary to rectify or complete the initial treatment [102].

- The decision between open surgery and endovascular repair may also be influenced by the level of expertise and preferences of the treating medical center, as well as by the resources and equipment available.

It should be emphasized that the treatment of traumatic aortic lesions must be highly personalized. Treatment strategies are developed following a comprehensive patient assessment, taking into account variables such as age, overall health, comorbidities and individual patient preferences. Treatment guidelines are continually evolving, reflecting technological advances and new evidence from clinical research.

VII- Course and prognosis of post-traumatic aortic injury :

Assessing the severity of trauma, in particular traumatic lesions of the aorta, and estimating patients' chances of survival are crucial aspects of medical management.

1-   Predictors of morbidity and mortality :

The management of patients undergoing surgery for traumatic aortic injury is complex, requiring in-depth assessment of factors predictive of morbidity and mortality.

The medical literature highlights the influence of the type of surgical procedure on post-operative complications [16, 88]. Endovascular techniques, which are less invasive, have been shown to reduce the risk of immediate complications such as major bleeding or infection. In contrast, open surgery, although more invasive, remains a relevant option in certain clinical situations, despite its association with higher rates of complications such as infections and respiratory problems.

Other studies emphasize the importance of factors such as patient age, comorbidities, time from trauma to hospital arrival, and time from hospital arrival to operation [47]. Pre-operative clinical data, in particular ISS and transfusion requirements, are particularly significant. An ISS greater than 30, indicating severe injury, is strongly associated with an increased risk of morbidity and mortality [104]. Similarly, transfusion requirements, notably the need to transfuse more than 4 units of red blood cells within 24 hours of surgery, reflect significant blood loss and hemodynamic instability, thus increasing the risk of complications. In addition, a ratio of fresh frozen plasma to red blood cells of less than 1: 1.5 is another worrying indicator, suggesting potential coagulopathy and a deteriorated clinical state [105].

In addition to factors directly related to the patient, several other elements play a crucial role in the outcome of surgical interventions for traumatic aortic lesions. Firstly, the experience and skill of the surgical team [106], particularly in endovascular or open surgical procedures, are decisive factors in the success of the operation.

An experienced team can better anticipate and manage potential complications, thus improving surgical outcomes. Secondly, the length of the operation

surgery also influences outcomes [107]. Prolonged procedures are often correlated with an increased risk of complications, including infectious complications, due to prolonged exposure and the increased complexity of the procedure. Thirdly, the specific techniques and devices used during surgery can affect the risk of complications [108]. Choosing the most appropriate technique for each specific case is essential to minimize risk.

The post-operative phase is also a vital aspect of management [109]. Effective pain management, rigorous infection prevention and careful monitoring of cardiovascular and pulmonary function are essential to reduce post-operative complications.

Finally, rehabilitation and regular follow-up play an important role in preventing long-term complications.

This comprehensive understanding of the various predictive factors is crucial to optimize surgical strategies and improve post-operative care, in order to reduce morbidity and mortality in patients with traumatic aortic injury.

2-   Complications of post-traumatic aortic injury :

2- 1- Early complications :

The early complications associated with surgery to treat traumatic aortic injury show notable variability, depending on the approach adopted. Each method carries specific risks and potential complications that deserve careful consideration:

Early complications of endovascular treatment are [20, 40]:

- Vascular access lesions and stent-related complications: Vascular lesions may occur at the stent insertion site, such as the formation of hematomas or false aneurysms. Migration or displacement of the stent (3%), as well as endoleak (2%), are significant risks.

- Endoleaks also represent a critical complication. They are classified into five distinct types [110], each reflecting a particular mechanism, which has important implications for the management and subsequent treatment of the condition. Detection and diagnosis of these leaks are usually performed with the aid of post-operative imaging examinations, such as computed tomography or thoracic angio-tomodensitometry.

- Neurological complications: spinal ischemia and paraplegia can result from obstruction of the artery supplying the spinal cord.

There is also a risk of stroke, particularly if debris is released into the bloodstream.

- Cardiac complications: Heart failure can occur if the heart is forced to pump through altered circulatory dynamics following stent placement. Although rare, myocardial infarction can also occur, often as a result of stress to the heart or embolism.

- Acute renal failure: This is a possible complication, linked to iodinated contrast media or hypoperfusion during the procedure.

Complications of open surgery are varied and may include [47]:

- Complications associated with incision and manipulation of the aorta, such as bleeding, hematoma or wound infection.

- Pulmonary complications such as pulmonary embolism, pneumonia or atelectasis, often due to prolonged intubation.

- Neurological complications: an increased risk of paraplegia or paresis, often caused by ischemia of the spinal cord during aortic occlusion.

- Cardiac complications: myocardial infarction, cardiac arrhythmias and congestive heart failure.

- Renal failure: may result from prolonged hypotension, or from the use of nephrotoxic drugs during the operation.

- Gastrointestinal problems: Mesenteric ischemia if the repair involves the area of the superior mesenteric artery.

- Crucially, advances in surgical techniques and post-operative care have helped to reduce the rate of these complications. Careful pre-operative risk management, together with rigorous post-operative follow-up, remains essential to minimize the risk of complications in both surgical approaches.

2- 2- Late complications :

Medium-term results of open repair and endovascular repair generally show a low rate of complications such as endoleaks, stent migration or the need for reinterventions, with an average follow-up period of 52 to 60 months, while data concerning long-term results remain, to date, insufficient [40].

Adapting follow-up protocols to include regular angioscan assessments can help detect and intervene early on complications, improving long-term outcomes.

At three months, the vast majority of our patients retained their stents without major complications, with the exception of a single patient who required a second stent because of a type I endoleak.

The same patient died a year later of a major complication after emergency reoperation. This case highlights the need for continued vigilance and perhaps a reassessment of follow-up criteria and endoleak management strategies.

These results confirm the feasibility and relative safety of endovascular intervention for the treatment of aortic lesions, while underscoring the need for careful monitoring and management of complications to optimize long-term results.

In the case of open aortic surgery, various late complications may arise [47]. These include the formation of false-channel aneurysms, resulting from persistent weakness of the aortic wall. Prosthetic infections are another serious complication that may require further surgical intervention. In addition, cardiac complications may arise, either as a result of deterioration in cardiac function, or as a direct consequence of the operation.

Finally, healing problems at the surgical incision can also occur, leading to delays in the healing process.

In the case of stent repairs, various late complications may also arise [111]. These include endoleaks, which may require corrective interventions. Stent migration, where the stent moves from its original position, can compromise its effectiveness. Stent thrombosis, which is the formation of blood clots inside the stent, can also lead to stent failure.

the stent, can obstruct blood flow. Finally, material fatigue, where wear or degradation of the stent material occurs over time, is another concern [90].

At our annual follow-up, it is notable that the majority of patients who underwent endovascular intervention showed satisfactory clinical outcomes, with the notable exception of one case of stent graft thrombosis, which was effectively managed with antiplatelet therapy. This observation underlines the relevance and efficacy of the endovascular approach to the treatment of aortic pathologies, while recognizing the need for ongoing vigilance to identify and treat potential complications such as thrombosis. On the other hand, the absence of complications in patients opting for open surgery contrasts with the risks associated with endovascular procedures, highlighting the relative safety of open surgery. However, this comparison also reveals the inherent advantages and disadvantages of each treatment method, requiring individualized assessment to choose the most appropriate option based on each patient's specific risk profile and conditions. These findings invite further discussion of follow-up protocols and complication prevention strategies, underlining the importance of informed therapeutic choice and rigorous post-operative management to optimize long-term results and minimize risks to patients.

2-   3- Complications s of non-operative RTA treatment:

The non-operative management of ALR presents a complex field with limited data on long-term outcomes [40].

Recently, a systematic review focusing on the non-operative management of ATN revealed a low percentage of critical aortic events [98]. However, this study also demonstrated significant lesion progression in 7.6% of cases, while lesion healing or improvement was recorded in 34% of patients. These data were collected over an extended follow-up period, ranging from 1 day to 118 months. It is important to note that when injury progression is noted on repeated imaging examinations, patients usually undergo surgical repair [98, 112].

This indicates that, although non-operative management may be a viable option for some low-grade ATR, careful monitoring is imperative to detect any signs of disease progression.

3-   Prognostic scores for post-traumatic aortic injury :

Several studies have analyzed the effectiveness and relevance of various prognostic scores. These include the Revised Trauma Score (RTS) and the Injury Severity Score (ISS), which are frequently used to quantify injury severity, guide resuscitation and establish surgical decisions [113].

4- Mortality in post-traumatic aortic injury:

Short-term mortality with endovascular treatment of AVR is lower than with conventional surgery.

The rate of complications associated with these endovascular methods is considerably reduced. The efficacy of this approach is supported by data from a rigorous meta-analysis including seven comparative studies between EVT and open surgery.

In a meta-analysis, Lettinga-van de Poll et al [20] found a significant difference in 30-day mortality rates between the two treatment modalities. While the open surgery group recorded a mortality rate of 18.9%, this rate was significantly lower, at 4%, in patients treated with VTE.

These results underline not only the short-term efficacy of VTE as the preferred treatment for AVR, but also its potential to minimize patient risk compared with more invasive methods such as conventional open surgery.

Open surgery, considered a conventional method for treating aortic lesions, is invasive and associated with a high risk of immediate post-operative complications. This may be attributed to the complexity of the lesions, the fragility of the aortic structure following trauma, or other operative risk factors.

Aortic stenting represents a less invasive approach with the potential for faster recovery and less pain for patients.

5- Determinants of posttraumatic survival of the aorta:

To examine the various factors influencing long-term survival after traumatic aortic rupture, the work of Arthurs et al. [114] and Deree et al.
[115] represent notable contributions in this field, highlighting the significant impact of aortic repair and the correlation between survival and several clinical variables such as shock, acidosis, and aortic lesion location. These studies

suggest that prompt and adequate surgical intervention, as well as early management of risk factors, are crucial to improving survival outcomes in patients with traumatic injuries to the thoracic aorta.

More recently, the study by Shiban et al (2021) [116] added a further dimension to this understanding by applying machine learning techniques to predict survival following traumatic aortic injury, highlighting the predictive role of comorbidities, particularly cardiac history, Glasgow Coma Scale score and the efficacy of thoracic endovascular aortic repair in survivors. In addition, factors such as smoking, pneumonia, and urinary tract infections were identified as negatively influencing survival, underlining the importance of comprehensive patient management beyond the aortic lesion alone.

Particularly revealing is the finding of a significant difference in survival according to the scannographic severity grade of aortic lesions. This indicates the crucial importance of accurate diagnostic imaging and lesion classification in therapeutic decision-making.

6- Patient follow-up and prevention of complications :

Follow-up protocols for patients treated for traumatic aortic injury with VTE or open surgery differ [10, 40, 93, 117, 118].

6- 1- Follow-up after endovascular treatment (EVT) :

- **Clinical monitoring:** Regular consultations with a vascular surgeon or cardiologist are essential to assess the patient's overall health, including management of cardiovascular risk factors.

- **Risk factor management**: Controlling hypertension and cholesterol, and stopping smoking are crucial. Medications such as statins or anti-hypertensives can be prescribed.

It is worth noting that, in one series observed [12], all patients who benefited from VTE were put on antiplatelet therapy.

- **Radiological checks:** Patients receive a contrast-enhanced CT scan before discharge to assess the position and integrity of the stent.

Frequent radiological checks are carried out in the first months after surgery, at 1, 3 and 6 months.

If the patient's condition is stable and without abnormalities, the frequency of radiological checks can be reduced. Clinical guidelines from the Society of Vascular Surgeons (SVS) suggest monitoring every 2 to 5 years [98].

6- 2- Follow-up after open surgery :

- **Immediate post-operative follow-up:** This phase focuses onmonitoring potential complications such as infections, scarring problems and pulmonary or cardiac complications.

- **Clinical monitoring:** Regular clinical monitoring is necessary to monitor overall recovery and manage cardiovascular risk factors.

- **Rehabilitation and lifestyle:** Rehabilitation may be necessary to regain strength and stamina, and lifestyle recommendations such as a healthy diet, smoking cessation and regular exercise are crucial.

- **Long-term radiological monitoring:** Although less frequent than with VTE, periodic CT or ultrasound examinations may be recommended.

- **Specific and personalized considerations:** It is essential to recognize that these monitoring protocols may vary according to individual factors such as patient age, comorbidities, type of aortic lesion and individual response to treatment. A personalized approach is therefore essential.

VIII-   Conclusion:

Since the 1950s, there has been considerable progress in the management of thoracic trauma and aortic lesions. Once treated mainly by open surgery, modern techniques now favor less invasive and safer endovascular repair, responding to the challenges posed by the frequency, severity and complexity of these lesions, often located at the level of the aortic isthmus.

Understanding aortic trauma highlights the need to refine the management and treatment of polytrauma patients. It is important for clinical practice, and drives further investigation of diagnostic and therapeutic approaches in this evolving field.

IX- Bibliography :

[1] Mathiot SP. Traumatic ruptures of the aortic isthmus 2000.

[2] Procházka V, Roman J, Jaluvka F, Jonszta T, Vrtková A, Pleva L, et al. Endovascular Repair of Thoracic Aorta Injury: 17 Years of Single-Center Experience. Med Sci Monit 2021;27.

[3] Steuer J, Björck M, Sonesson B, Resch T, Dias N, Hultgren R, et al. Editor's Choice - Durability of Endovascular Repair in Blunt Traumatic Thoracic Aortic Injury: Long-Term Outcome from Four Tertiary Referral Centers. Eur J Vasc Endovasc Surg Off J Eur Soc Vasc Surg 2015;50:460-5.

[4] Hiller RJ, Mikocka-Walus AA, Cameron PA. Aortic transection: demographics, treatment and outcomes in Victoria, Australia. Emerg Med J EMJ 2010;27:368-71.

[5] Fabian TC, Richardson JD, Croce MA, Smith JS, Rodman G, Kearney PA, et al. Prospective study of blunt aortic injury: Multicenter Trial of the American Association for the Surgery of Trauma. J Trauma 1997;42:374-80; discussion 380- 383.

[6] Jamieson WRE, Janusz MT, Gudas VM, Burr LH, Fradet GJ, Henderson C. Traumatic rupture of the thoracic aorta: third decade of experience. Am J Surg 2002;183:571-5.

[7] Zoulati M, Bakkali T, Aghoutane N, Lyazidi Y, Chtata H, Taberkant M. Acute post-traumatic dissection of the descending thoracic aorta. JMV-J Médecine Vasc 2019;44:367-73.

[8] Jahromi AS, Kazemi K, Safar HA, Doobay B, Cinà CS. Traumatic rupture of the thoracic aorta: cohort study and systematic review. J Vasc Surg 2001;34:1029-34.

[9] Cardarelli MG, McLaughlin JS, Downing SW, Brown JM, Attar S,

Griffith BP. Management of traumatic aortic rupture: a 30-year experience. Ann Surg 2002;236:465-9; discussion 469-470.

[10] Lee WA, Matsumura JS, Mitchell RS, Farber MA, Greenberg RK, Azizzadeh A, et al. Endovascular repair of traumatic thoracic aortic injury: clinical practice guidelines of the Society for Vascular Surgery. J Vasc Surg 2011;53:187-92.

[11] Xenos ES, Abedi NN, Davenport DL, Minion DJ, Hamdallah O, Sorial EE, et al. Meta-analysis of endovascular vs open repair for traumatic descending thoracic aortic rupture. J Vasc Surg 2008;48:1343-51.

[12] Denguir R, Frikha I, Kaouel K, Abdennadher M, Ziadi J, Jemel A, et al. Management of post-traumatic aortic isthmus ruptures. About 37 cases. J Mal Vasc 2013;38:13-21.

[13] Dake MD, Patel HJ. Thoracic Branch Endoprosthesis: Early Case Experience and the Clinical Trial n.d.

[14] Greendyke RM. Traumatic rupture of aorta; special reference to automobile accidents. JAMA 1966;195:527-30.

[15] Cook J, Salerno C, Krishnadasan B, Nicholls S, Meissner M, Karmy-Jones R. The effect of changing presentation and management on the outcome of blunt rupture of the thoracic aorta. J Thorac Cardiovasc Surg 2006;131:594-600.

[16] Cheng Y-T, Cheng C-T, Wang S-Y, Wu VC-C, Chu P-H, Chou A-H, et al. Long-term Outcomes of Endovascular and Open Repair for Traumatic Thoracic Aortic Injury. JAMA Netw Open 2019;2:e187861.

[17] Rousseau H, Dambrin C, Marcheix B, Richeux L, Mazerolles M, Cron C, et al. Acute traumatic aortic rupture: A comparison of surgical and stentgraft repair. J Thorac Cardiovasc Surg 2005;129:1050-5.

[18] Gammie JS, Shah AS, Hattler BG, Kormos RL, Peitzman AB, Griffith BP, et al. Traumatic aortic rupture: diagnosis and management. Ann Thorac Surg 1998;66:1295-300.

[19] Akowuah E, Baumbach A, Wilde P, Angelini G, Bryan AJ. Emergency repair of traumatic aortic rupture: endovascular versus conventional open repair. J Thorac Cardiovasc Surg 2007;134:897-901.

[20] Lettinga-van De Poll T, Schurink GWH, De Haan MW, Verbruggen JPAM, Jacobs MJ. Endovascular treatment of traumatic rupture of the thoracic aorta. Br J Surg 2007;94:525-33.

[21] Dinh K, Limmer A, Ngai C, Cho T, Young N, Hsu J. Blunt thoracic aorta injuries, an Australian single center's perspective. ANZ J Surg 2021;91:662-7.

[22] Bae M, Jeon CH, Kwon H, Kim JH, Choi SU, Song S. Evaluation of Zone 2 Thoracic Endovascular Aortic Repair Performed with and without Prophylactic Embolization of the Left Subclavian Artery in Patients with Traumatic Aortic Injury. Korean J Radiol 2021;22:577.

[23] Trachiotis GD, Sell JE, Pearson GD, Martin GR, Midgley FM. Traumatic Thoracic Aortic Rupture in the Pediatric Patient. Ann Thorac Surg 1996;62:724-32.

[24] Noly P-E, Mercier O, Angel C, Fabre D, Mussot S, Brenot P, et al. Treatment of traumatic ruptures of the aortic isthmus in 2014. J Eur Urgences Réanimation 2015;27:161-71.

[25] Sun J, Ren K, Zhang L, Xue C, Duan W, Liu J, et al. Traumatic blunt thoracic aortic injury: a 10-year single-center retrospective analysis. J Cardiothorac Surg 2022;17:335.

[26] Asgarzadeh M, Fischer D, Verma SK, Courtney TK, Christiani DC. The impact of weather, road surface, time-of-day, and light conditions on severity

of bicycle- motor vehicle crash injuries. Am J Ind Med 2018;61:556-65.

[27] Richens D. The mechanism of injury in blunt traumatic rupture of the aorta. Eur J Cardiothorac Surg 2002;21:288-93.

[28] Gaffey AC, Zhang J, Saka E, Quatromoni JG, Glaser J, Kim P, et al. Natural History of Nonoperative Management of Grade II Blunt Thoracic Aortic Injury. Ann Vasc Surg 2020;65:124-9.

[29] Ayella RJ, Hankins JR, Turney SZ, Cowley RA. Ruptured thoracic aorta due to blunt trauma: J Trauma Inj Infect Crit Care 1977;17:199-205.

[30] Cowley RA, Turney SZ, Hankins JR, Rodriguez A, Attar S, Shankar BS. Rupture of thoracic aorta caused by blunt trauma. A fifteen-year experience. J Thorac Cardiovasc Surg 1990;100:652-60; discussion 660661.

[31] Stemper BD, Yoganandan N, Pintar FA, Brasel KJ. Multiple Subfailures Characterize Blunt Aortic Injury: J Trauma Inj Infect Crit Care 2007;62:1171-4.

[32] Igiebor OS, Waseem M. Aortic Trauma. StatPearls, Treasure Island (FL): StatPearls Publishing; 2023.

[33] Goarin JP, Barbry T. Traumatic lesions of the aorta n.d.

[34] Patel NR, Dick E, Batrick N, Jenkins M, Kashef E. Pearls and pitfalls in imaging of blunt traumatic thoracic aortic injury: a pictorial review. Br J Radiol 2018:20180130.

[35] Teixeira PGR, Inaba K, Barmparas G, Georgiou C, Toms C, Noguchi TT, et al. Blunt Thoracic Aortic Injuries: An Autopsy Study. J Trauma Inj Infect Crit Care 2011;70:197-202.

[36] Schulman CI, Carvajal D, Lopez PP, Soffer D, Habib F, Augenstein J. Incidence and Crash Mechanisms of Aortic Injury During the Past Decade. J Trauma Inj Infect Crit Care 2007;62:664-7.

[37] Demetriades D, Velmahos GC, Scalea TM, Jurkovich GJ, Karmy-Jones R, Teixeira PG, et al. Operative Repair or Endovascular Stent Graft in Blunt Traumatic

Thoracic Aortic Injuries: Results of an American Association for the Surgery of Trauma Multicenter Study. J Trauma Inj Infect Crit Care 2008;64:561-71.

[38] Lesèche G, Alsac J-M, Castier Y. Acute post-traumatic rupture of the aortic isthmus. J Chir (Paris) 2008;145:115-21.

[39] De Mestral C, Dueck A, Sharma SS, Haas B, Gomez D, Hsiao M, et al. Evolution of the Incidence, Management, and Mortality of Blunt Thoracic Aortic Injury: A Population-Based Analysis. J Am Coll Surg 2013;216:1110-5.

[40] Isselbacher EM, Preventza O, Hamilton Black J, Augoustides JG, Beck AW, Bolen MA, et al. 2022 ACC/AHA Guideline for the Diagnosis and Management of Aortic Disease: A Report of the American Heart Association/American College of Cardiology Joint Committee on Clinical Practice Guidelines. Circulation 2022;146.

[41] Classification of Blunt Traumatic Aortic Injury. n.d.

[42] Feczko JD, Lynch L, Pless JE, Clark MA, McClain J, Hawley DA. An autopsy case review of 142 nonpenetrating (blunt) injuries of the aorta: J Trauma Inj Infect Crit Care 1992;33:846- 9.

[43] Townend JN, Davies MK, Jones EL. Fatal rupture of an unsuspected posttraumatic aneurysm of the thoracic aorta during pregnancy. Heart 1991;66:248- 9.

[44] Parmley LF, Mattingly TW, Manion WC, Jahnke EJ. Nonpenetrating Traumatic Injury of the Aorta. Circulation 1958;17:1086-101.

[45] Hudson HM, Woodson J, Hirsch E. The Management of Traumatic Aortic Tear in the Multiply-Injured Patient. Ann Vasc Surg 1991;5:445-8.

[46] Nzewi O, Slight RD, Zamvar V. Management of Blunt Thoracic Aortic Injury. Eur J Vasc Endovasc Surg 2006;31:18-27.

[47] Chiba K, Abe H, Kitanaka Y, Miyairi T, Makuuchi H. Conventional surgical repair of traumatic rupture of the thoracic aorta. Gen Thorac Cardiovasc Surg 2014;62:713-9.

[48] Fox N, Schwartz D, Salazar JH, Haut ER, Dahm P, Black JH, et al. Evaluation and management of blunt traumatic aortic injury: A practice management guideline from the Eastern Association for the Surgery of Trauma. J Trauma Acute Care Surg 2015;78:136-46.

[49] Rodriguez-Merchán EC, Rubio-Suárez JC, editors. Complex fractures ofthe limbs: diagnosis and management. Cham Heidelberg: Springer; 2014.

[50] Kaewlai R, De Moya MA, Santos A, Asrani AV, Avery LL, Novelline RA. Blunt Cardiac Injury in Trauma Patients with Thoracic Aortic Injury. Emerg Med Int 2011;2011:1-6.

[51] Emet M, Akoz A, Aslan S, Saritas A, Cakir Z, Acemoglu H. Assessment of cardiac injury in patients with blunt chest trauma. Eur J Trauma Emerg Surg 2010;36:441-7.

[52] Nagy KK, Krosner SM, Roberts RR, Joseph KT, Smith RF, Barrett J. Determining Which Patients Require Evaluation for Blunt Cardiac Injury following Blunt Chest Trauma. World J Surg 2001;25:108-11.

[53] Gaul C, Dietrich W, Friedrich I, Sirch J, Erbguth FJ. Neurological Symptoms in Type A Aortic Dissections. Stroke 2007;38:292-7.

[54] Laforet EG. Acute hypertension as a diagnostic clue in traumatic rupture of the thoracic aorta. Am J Surg 1965;110:948-50.

[55] Fox S, Pierce WS, Waldhausen JA. Acute hypertension: Its significance in traumatic aortic rupture. J Thorac Cardiovasc Surg 1979;77:622-5.

[56] Sasamoto N, Akutsu K, Yamamoto T, Otsuka T, Sangen H, Hayashi H, et al. Characteristics of Inter-Arm Difference in Blood Pressure in Acute Aortic Dissection. J Nippon Med Sch 2021;88:467-74.

[57] Botz B, Bickle I. Focussed Assessment with Sonography for Trauma (FAST) scan. Radiopaedia.org, Radiopaedia.org; 2013.

[58] Schiavone WA, Ghumrawi BK, Catalano DR, Haver DW, Pipitone AJ, L'Hommedieu RH, et al. The use of echocardiography in the emergency management of nonpenetrating traumatic cardiac rupture. Ann Emerg Med 1991;20:1248-50.

[59] Byun CS, Park I, Kim T, Lee E, Oh J. Cardiac Rupture of the Junction of the Right Atrium and Superior Vena Cava in Blunt Thoracic Trauma. Korean J Crit Care Med 2015;30:27-30.

[60] O'Conor CE. Diagnosing traumatic rupture of the thoracic aorta in the emergency department. Emerg Med J EMJ 2004;21:414-9.

[61] Wintermark M, Wicky S, Schnyder P. Imaging of acute traumatic injuries of the thoracic aorta. Eur Radiol 2002;12:431-42.

[62] Ait Ali Yahia D, Bouvier A, Nedelcu C, Urdulashvili M, Thouveny F, Ridereau C, et al. Imaging of thoracic aortic injury. Diagn Interv Imaging 2015;96:79-88.

[63] Patel NH, Stephens KE, Mirvis SE, Shanmuganathan K, Mann FA. Imaging of acute thoracic aortic injury due to blunt trauma: a review. Radiology 1998;209:335- 48.

[64] Woodring JH. The normal mediastinum in blunt traumatic rupture of the thoracic aorta and brachiocephalic arteries. J Emerg Med 1990;8:467-76.

[65] Creasy JD, Chiles C, Routh WD, Dyer RB. Overview of traumatic injury of the thoracic aorta. RadioGraphics 1997;17:27-45.

[66] Heystraten F, Rosenbusch G, Kingma L, Lacquet L. Chronic posttraumatic aneurysm of the thoracic aorta: surgically correctable occult threat. Am J Roentgenol 1986;146:303-8.

[67] Johnson P, Anderson R, Gamble C, Van Bogaert E, Joshi J. Traumatic aortic injury from pellet gun: A case report. Radiol Case Rep 2023;18:1368-71.

[68] Mirvis SE, Shanmuganathan K, Buell J, Rodriguez A. Use of Spiral Computed Tomography for the Assessment of Blunt Trauma Patients with Potential Aortic Injury: J Trauma Inj Infect Crit Care 1998;45:922-30.

[69] Gavant ML. Helical CT grading of traumatic aortic injuries. Radiol Clin North Am 1999;37:553-74.

[70] Starnes BW, Lundgren RS, Gunn M, Quade S, Hatsukami TS, Tran NT, et al. A new classification scheme for treating blunt aortic injury. J Vasc Surg 2012;55:47- 54.

[71] Vignon P, Guéret P, Vedrinne JM, Lagrange P, Cornu E, Abrieu O, et al. Role of transesophageal echocardiography in the diagnosis and management of traumatic aortic disruption. Circulation 1995;92:2959-68.

[72] Chirillo F, Totis O, Cavarzerani A, Bruni A, Farnia A, Sarpellon M, et al. Usefulness of transthoracic and transoesophageal echocardiography in recognition and management of cardiovascular injuries after blunt chest trauma. Heart 1996;75:301-6.

[73] Fisher RG, Sanchez-Torres M, Thomas JW, Whigham CJ. Subtle or atypical injuries of the thoracic aorta and brachiocephalic vessels in blunt thoracic trauma. RadioGraphics 1997;17:835-49.

[74] DelRossi AJ, Cernaianu AC, Cilley JH, Madden L, Spence RK. Multiple Traumatic Disruptions of the Thoracic Aorta. Chest 1990;97:1307-9.

[75] Vivien B, Cluzel P, Riou B. Large-vessel thoracic injury due to

deceleration. EMC - Médecine Urgence 2009;4:1-9.

[76] Goarin J-P, Cluzel P, Gosgnach M, Lamine K, Coriat P, Riou B. Evaluation of Transesophageal Echocardiography for Diagnosis of Traumatic Aortic Injury. Anesthesiology 2000;93:1373-7.

[77] Hoffman JRH, Chowdhury R, Johnson LS, Brewster LP, Duwayri Y, Reeves JG, et al. Posttraumatic Resuscitation Affects Stent Graft Sizing in Patients with Blunt Thoracic Aortic Injury. Am Surg 2016;82:75-8.

[78] Calcaterra D. Blunt Traumatic Aortic Injury. In: Sözen S, Hakan Kanat B, editors. Trauma Emerg. Surg, IntechOpen; 2022.

[79] Dollery W, Driscoll P. Resuscitation after high energy polytrauma. Br Med Bull 1999;55:785-805.

[80] Warren RL, Akins CW, Conn AK, Hilgenberg AD, McCabe CJ. Acute traumatic disruption of the thoracic aorta: emergency department management. Ann Emerg Med 1992;21:391-6.

[81] Pate JW, Gavant ML, Weiman DS, Fabian TC. Traumatic rupture of the aortic isthmus: program of selective management. World J Surg 1999;23:59-63.

[82] Pontone G, Marano R, Agricola E, Alushi B, Bartorelli A, Cameli M, et al. Recommendations in pre-procedural imaging assessment for transcatheter aortic

valve implantation intervention: Italian Society of Cardiology (SIC)-Italian Society of Medical and Interventional Radiology (SIRM) position paper part 1 (Clinical Indication and Basic Technical Aspects, Heart Team, Role of Echocardiography). J Cardiovasc Med 2022;23:216-27.

[83] Akins CW, Buckley MJ, Daggett W, McIlduff JB, Austen WG. AcuteTraumatic Disruption of the Thoracic Aorta: A Ten-Year Experience.

AnnThorac Surg 1981;31:305-9.

[84] Bouchart F, Bessou JP, Tabley A, Litzler PY, Haas-Hubscher C, Redonnet M, et al. Acute traumatic ruptures of the thoracic aorta and its branches. Résultats du traitement chirurgical***Communication présentée à l'Académie nationale de chirurgie au cours de la séance du 22 mars 2000. Ann Chir 2001;126:201-11.

[85] Di Eusanio M, Folesani G, Berretta P, Petridis FD, Pantaleo A, Russo V, et al. Delayed Management of Blunt Traumatic Aortic Injury: Open Surgical Versus Endovascular Repair. Ann Thorac Surg 2013;95:1591-7.

[86] Alarhayem AQ, Rasmussen TE, Farivar B, Lim S, Braverman M, Hardy D, et al. Timing of repair of blunt thoracic aortic injuries in the thoracic endovascular aortic repair era. J Vasc Surg 2021;73:896-902.

[87] Holmes JH, Bloch RD, Hall RA, Carter YM, Karmy-Jones RC. Natural history of traumatic rupture of the thoracic aorta managed nonoperatively: a longitudinal analysis. Ann Thorac Surg 2002;73:1149-54.

[88] Alsac J-M, Boura B, Desgranges P, Fabiani J-N, Becquemin J-P, Leseche G. Immediate endovascular repair for acute traumatic injuries of the thoracic aorta: A multicenter analysis of 28 cases. J Vasc Surg 2008;48:1369-74.

[89] Melnitchouk S, Pfammatter T, Kadner A, Dave H, Witzke H, Trentz O, et al. Emergency stent-graft placement for hemorrhage control in acute thoracic aortic rupture1. Eur J Cardiothorac Surg 2004;25:1032-8.

[90] Kim SH, Huh U, Song S, Kim MS, Kim CW, Jeon CH, et al. Open repair versus thoracic endovascular aortic repair for treating traumatic aortic injury. Asian J Surg 2022;45:2224-30.

[91] Demers P, Miller C, Scott Mitchell R, Kee ST, Lynn Chagonjian RN, Dake MD. Chronic traumatic aneurysms of the descending thoracic aorta:

midterm results of endovascular repair using first and second-generation stent-grafts. Eur J Cardio- Thorac Surg Off J Eur Assoc Cardio-Thorac Surg 2004;25:394-400.

[92] Dorweiler B, Dueber C, Neufang A, Schmiedt W, Pitton MB, Oelert H. Endovascular treatment of acute bleeding complications in traumatic aortic rupture and aortobronchial fistula. Eur J Cardio-Thorac Surg Off J Eur Assoc Cardio-Thorac Surg 2001;19:739-45.

[93] Chalvatzoulis E, Megalopoulos A, Trellopoulos G, Ananiadou O, Papoulidis P, Kemanetzi I, et al. Endovascular repair of traumatic aortic transection. Interact Cardiovasc Thorac Surg 2010;11:238-42.

[94] Nano G, Mazzaccaro D, Malacrida G, Occhiuto MT, Stegher S, Tealdi DG. Delayed endovascular treatment of descending aorta stent graft collapse in a patient treated for post traumatic aortic rupture: a case report. J Cardiothorac Surg 2011;6:76.

[95] DuBose JJ, Leake SS, Brenner M, Pasley J, O'Callaghan T, Luo-Owen X, et al. Contemporary management and outcomes of blunt thoracic aortic injury: a multicenter retrospective study. J Trauma Acute Care Surg 2015;78:360-9.

[96] Fortuna GR, Perlick A, DuBose JJ, Leake SS, Charlton-Ouw KM, Miller CC, et al. Injury grade is a predictor of aortic-related death among patients with blunt thoracic aortic injury. J Vasc Surg 2016;63:1225-31.

[97] Pang D, Hildebrand D, Bachoo P. Thoracic endovascular repair (TEVAR) versus open surgery for blunt traumatic thoracic aortic injury. Cochrane Database Syst Rev 2015:CD006642.

[98] Kenel-Pierre S, Ramos Duran E, Abi-Chaker A, Melendez F, Alghamdi H, Bornak A, et al. The role of heparin in endovascular repair of blunt thoracic aortic injury. J Vasc Surg 2019;70:1809-15.

[99] Scalea TM, Feliciano DV, DuBose JJ, Ottochian M, O'Connor JV, Morrison JJ. Blunt Thoracic Aortic Injury: Endovascular Repair Is Now the Standard. J Am Coll Surg 2019;228:605-10.

[100] Murad MH, Rizvi AZ, Malgor R, Carey J, Alkatib AA, Erwin PJ, et al. Comparative effectiveness of the treatments for thoracic aortic transection. J Vasc Surg 2011;53:193-199.e1-21.

[101] AlSayyari T, Almatar Z, AlShomar A, Alnamshan M. Traumatic Thoracic Aortic Injury in a Three-Year-Old Patient: A Case Report. Cureus 2022.

[102] Dziekiewicz M, Laska G, Makowski K. Undersized Stentgraft Placement for Traumatic Descending Aorta Rupture, and What Is Next? Am J Case Rep 2020;21.

[103] Inaba Y, Iida Y, Oka H, Miki T, Hachiya T, Shimizu H. Blunt traumatic aortic injury to the brachiocephalic and left carotid arteries. Gen Thorac Cardiovasc Surg Cases 2022;1:11.

[104] Mohapatra A, Liang NL, Makaroun MS, Schermerhorn ML, Farber A, Eslami MH. Risk factors for mortality after endovascular repair for blunt thoracic aortic injury. J Vasc Surg 2020;71:768-73.

[105] Echeverria AB, Branco BC, Goshima KR, Hughes JD, Mills JL. Outcomes of endovascular management of acute thoracic aortic emergencies in an academic level 1 trauma center. Am J Surg 2014;208:974-80; discussion 979-980.

[106] Dake MD, White RA, Diethrich EB, Greenberg RK, Criado FJ, Bavaria JE, et al. Report on endograft management of traumatic thoracic aortic transections at 30 days and 1 year from a multidisciplinary subcommittee of the Society for Vascular Surgery Outcomes Committee. J Vasc Surg 2011;53:1091-6.

[107] Buz S, Zipfel B, Mulahasanovic S, Pasic M, Weng Y, Hetzer R. Conventional surgical repair and endovascular treatment of acute traumatic aortic rupture☆. Eur J Cardiothorac Surg 2008;33:143-9.

[108] Kasirajan K, Heffernan D, Langsfeld M. Acute Thoracic Aortic Trauma: A Comparison of Endoluminal Stent Grafts with Open Repair and Nonoperative Management. Ann Vasc Surg 2003;17:589-95.

[109] Schraag S. Postoperative management. Best Pract Res Clin Anaesthesiol 2016;30:381-93.

[110] Heye S. Diagnosis and treatment of endoleaks after endovascular repair of thoracic and abdominal aortic aneurysms. JBR-BTR Organ Soc R Belge Radiol SRBR Orgaan Van K Belg Ver Voor Radiol KBVR 2013;96:189-95.

[111] Martin C, Thony F, Rodiere M, Bouzat P, Lavagne P, Durand M, et al. Long- term results following emergency stent graft repair for traumatic rupture of the aortic

isthmus. Eur J Cardio-Thorac Surg Off J Eur Assoc Cardio-Thorac Surg 2017;51:767-72.

[112] Pang D, Hildebrand D, Bachoo P. Thoracic endovascular repair (TEVAR) versus open surgery for blunt traumatic thoracic aortic injury. Cochrane Database Syst Rev 2019;2:CD006642.

[113] Massaga F, Washington LA, Ngayomela IH, Mwami AS, Shabhay A.n Management of a road traffic accident poly-trauma patient in a limited regional resource hospital setting in Tanzania: Review of literature and case report. Int J Surg Case Rep 2023;110:108764.

[114] Arthurs ZM, Starnes BW, Sohn VY, Singh N, Martin MJ, Andersen CA. Functional and survival outcomes in traumatic blunt thoracic aortic injuries: An analysis of the National Trauma Databank. J Vasc Surg

2009;49:988-94.

[115] Deree J, Shenvi E, Fortlage D, Stout P, Potenza B, Hoyt DB, et al. Patient factors and operating room resuscitation predict mortality in traumatic abdominal aortic injury: A 20-year analysis. J Vasc Surg 2007;45:493-7.

[116] Shiban N, Gaul J, Zhan H, Elhabr A, Kokabi N, Johnson J-O, et al. Machine Learning Methods to Predict Survival in Patients Following Traumatic Aortic Injury. Health Informatics; 2021.

[117] Asaid R, Boyce G, Atkinson N. Endovascular Repair of Acute Traumatic Aortic Injury: Experience of a Level-1 Trauma Center. Ann Vasc Surg 2014;28:1391-5.

[118] Kaneyuki D, Asakura T, Iguchi A, Yoshitake A, Tokunaga C, Tochii M, et al. Early- and long-term results of thoracic endovascular aortic repair for blunt traumatic
thoracic aortic injury: a single-centre experience. Eur J Cardiothorac Surg 2019;56:307-12.

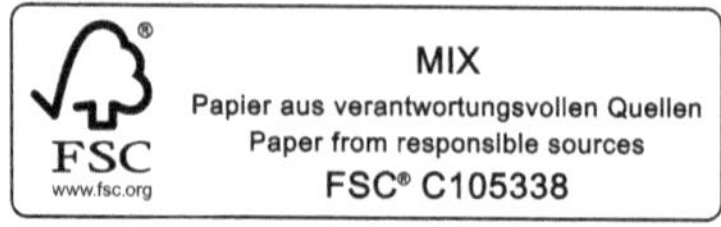

Printed by Books on Demand GmbH, Norderstedt / Germany